Dash Diet

The Comprehensive Cookbook To Boost Metabolism And
Lose Weight Efficiently While Maintaining Heart Health

*(Increase Your Metabolism And Enhance Your Health
While Reducing Your Blood Pressure)*

Theodore Hartman

TABLE OF CONTENT

Chapter 1: Benefits Of The Dash Diet

In recent years, a great deal of attention has been paid to the quantity of salt present in prepackaged and processed foods. It has been estimated that approximately 710 % of our daily salt intake originates from these foods in a standard diet. This can often result in individuals unknowingly consuming perilously high levels of sodium daily. Changing to a low-sodium diet becomes a goal for a large number of individuals, but a necessity for others.

In order to reduce blood pressure, the American College of Cardiology recommends low sodium diets for the treatment of mild hypertension. The DASH regimen is just such a regimen.

As the name implies, a low sodium diet is intended to reduce sodium intake to approximately half of what would be anticipated from a typical daily diet. In conjunction with a low-sodium diet, diuretics are frequently used to relieve the body of excess fluid retention. In this manner, they can be beneficial for weight loss.

The DASH Diet is designed to be simple to follow, so it can readily become a part of a permanent and healthier lifestyle change. Contrary to popular belief, a person on this type of diet has access to an abundance of food options, so the food they consume does not have to be dull and tasteless. In fact, if fresh produce is your primary source, the food you consume will likely appear and taste much fresher and more vibrant than you may have been accustomed to previously.

Chapter 2: The Beginning Of The Dash Diet

With so many diets available, you may be wondering why you should choose the DASH diet. This diet is not a novelty diet, which is the primary reason why so many individuals choose it. Diets are not designed to last a lifetime, so many people fail to adhere to them. These regimens promoted by the mainstream media may be effective, but only temporarily. They were never intended to be maintained. In reality, the majority of people who lose weight on this diet acquire it back within a few years. Dietary Approaches to Stop Hypertension (DASH) aims to alter your lifestyle so that you remain healthy for a lifetime.

Did you know that approximately fifty million Americans suffer from hypertension? This number is somewhere around 2 billion worldwide! Scientists discovered a direct correlation between high blood pressure and a variety of cardiovascular diseases. This means that if your blood pressure is excessive, you have a greater chance of suffering from a stroke, heart failure, heart attack, and even kidney disease. This is particularly true for those between the ages of 8 0 and 70 who have hypertension. In response to the prevalence of hypertension in the United States, the National Institutes of Health chose to take action.

DASH Diet Experiment

After the scientist discovered this connection, it was time to evaluate the diets. In the experiment, three distinct cuisines were chosen. One of these diets was selected as the control diet, which consisted of a diet with average amounts of fiber, magnesium, calcium, and potassium, as well as fat and protein. In comparison to the control group, the first experimental diet contained a greater quantity of fruits and vegetables. This indicates that the magnesium and potassium levels were intended to exceed the average U.S. consumption at the time. Along with this diet came an increase in fiber content. The second diet was also rich in fruits and vegetables, but includes low-fat dairy products selectively, resulting in a diet that is lower in saturated fat and higher in protein and fiber. This second regimen became known as the DASH diet.

Today's DASH diet emphasizes whole grains, legumes, fish, and poultry. Additionally, it contains fewer desserts, red meats, and processed foods. With the addition of healthier items, the diet reaches the 710 th percentile for nutrients in the United States. This diet is exceptionally abundant in calcium, magnesium, and potassium. The nutrients played a significant role in lowering blood pressure and, as a secondary effect, aid in weight loss!

Instead of focusing on a single nutrient, the entire dietary pattern was evaluated for the DASH diet, which was one of its most distinctive features. In addition to lowering blood pressure, the DASH diet includes many anti-oxidant-rich foods that aid and prevent other chronic conditions. According to some studies, this diet can help reduce or prevent diseases like stroke, heart disease, and cancer. Additionally, it was useful for preventing kidney stones. Where can you possibly go wrong? It is not surprising that the DASH diet is highly regarded by many dietitians and physicians.

At the conclusion of the investigation, it was determined that the DASH diet did indeed affect blood pressure in individuals with moderate to severe hypertension. With the aid of the DASH diet, these individuals were able to reduce their systolic and diastolic blood pressure by an average of 10 .10 mm. Obviously, this contrasts with the control diet, which was designed to parody the modern, average American diet. It was discovered that subjects who ingested more fruits and vegetables were more likely to reduce their blood pressure effectively. These results were observed as early as two weeks after beginning the regimen.

Chapter 3: The Dash Diet Recommendations

Dietary Approaches to Stop Hypertension (DASH) is one healthful eating plan. It is a lifetime approach to healthful eating intended to prevent or treat hypertension (high blood pressure). It also aids in weight loss, although this is not its primary function. It emphasizes eating a variety of foods, obtaining the proper quantity of nutrients, and consuming the appropriate portion sizes.

The diet promotes sodium reduction by allowing you to consume a variety of foods abundant in blood pressure-lowering nutrients such as magnesium, calcium, and potassium. The main purpose of the diet is to allow you to reduce your sodium intake, thereby lowering your blood pressure and enhancing your health.

In two weeks, you may reduce your blood pressure if you adopt the DASH diet. As you become accustomed to the DASH diet, your systolic blood pressure may decrease by 8 to 2 8 points. In addition to moderating blood pressure, the diet follows the dietary guidelines for preventing cancer, osteoporosis, cardiovascular disease, diabetes, and stroke.

The focus is on Sodium

Many individuals develop elevated blood pressure due to a diet high in sodium. Sodium retains water in the body, which causes the pulse to beat faster. The heart transports sodium throughout the blood vessels as it circulates blood. This activity raises the arterial pressure.

Sodium is primarily consumed in the form of salt. The mineral is also naturally present in some foods. However, the most significant contributor to elevated blood pressure is the sodium added to restaurant and processed foods. Adding salt from a salt shaker to food also causes hypertension.

Experts concur that adhering to the DASH diet can aid in lowering blood pressure. The DASH diet meal plan makes it simpler to consume less salty foods because the diet has a significantly lower sodium content than the typical American diet. The DASH diet also contains various other nutrients that aid in blood pressure regulation.

Tips for Sodium Reduction

The following chapter discusses a two-phase implementation strategy for the DASH diet. However, once you've effectively completed the two phases of the diet, you can follow the tips below.

Consume more organic foods and fewer processed foods high in sodium.

Reduce your salt intake gradually, and your taste buds will eventually acclimate.

Make an effort to recreate some of your beloved restaurant dishes at home. When you cook at home, you have control over the amount of salt used.

Choose fish, skinless poultry, lean fresh meats, tuna in water-packed cans, and eggs over processed meats, cured meats, and canned foods high in sodium.

Instead of salt, contribute flavor. Enhance the flavor of your dishes with salt-free seasoning blends, such as vinegar, citrus, lemon, spices, and herbs.

Restrict your consumption of refined, high-sodium convenience foods:

- Sauces such as soy sauce, barbecue sauce, and ketchup

- Vegetables, broth, and dishes in a can

- Snack foods such as potato crisps, salted pretzels, and crackers

- Packaged flavored pasta, grain, and rice mixtures

- Pizza and prepared dinners

Before adding salt, sample the food first. Get rid of the salt shaker if you are tempted to sprinkle salt on your food.

Choose low-sodium broths, soups, vegetable liquids, vegetables in a can, soy sauce, and other condiments.

To ascertain the sodium content of processed or packaged foods, consult the food labels (Nutrition Facts). With some planning, you can still incorporate these nutrients into your diet. Consume foods containing 8 80 mg or more of sodium per serving sparingly.

Nutritional Data

Everyone is familiar with the appearance of a 'Nutrition Facts' label, as it is present on all industrialized and packaged foods. It also serves as a guide for reducing your sodium intake. According to studies, individuals who pay attention to the 'Nutrition Facts' label are healthier than those who disregard it.

Examine the Sodium

The sodium content is listed in milligrams on the label. It can also be expressed as a percentage of the daily value. In the DASH diet, you should not consume more than 2,6 00 milligrams of sodium per day. Examine the percentage of daily value. If the sodium content is below 10 % of the DV, the food is minimal in sodium. If 20% or more of the DV is sodium, the food is high in sodium.

Check the Container Servings and Serving Size

Nutritional information, including sodium content, is based on serving size. However, the serving measurement is not always the amount consumed. If the portion size is lesser or larger than the listed serving size, the sodium must be calculated accordingly.

What Ingredients are Includcd?

The Nutrition Facts label includes the ingredient list, which is typically located beneath the label. If sodium-rich ingredients are listed first, it is likely that the food item has a high sodium content. Even if the salty ingredient is buried in the ingredient list, you should still verify the sodium content of each serving.

Learn the Language of Labels

Labels are typically located on frozen dinner packages, cracker cases, and soup can fronts. The sodium content can be found on the product labels. While "reduced sodium" may sound healthful, the actual sodium content may exceed your daily sodium limit. Here are some sodium claims defined by the U.S. Food and Drug Administration (FDA).

Or less than 6 10 milligrams of sodium

No salt added, unsalted - There is no salt applied during processing.

Sodium- and salt-free - Less than 10 mg per serving

Low sodium - less than 2 8 0 mg

Reduced sodium - 210 % less sodium than the standard product.

Light in sodium - containing 10 0% less sodium than the standard version

Compare the 'Nutrition Facts' labels of two similar products in the grocery store. Identify the culinary item with the lowest sodium content.

Behind the DASH Diet

Originally, the DASH diet was intended to be a heart-healthy solution. The original diet from the 2 990s adhered to the recommendation of consuming a high amount of carbohydrates. The original diet also recommended a reduced fat intake and asserted that people consumed an excessive amount of protein. Possibly due to such recommendations, the "diabetes epidemic" emerged.

The revised DASH diet enables individuals to take advantage of newer research on the advantages of a reduced intake of added sugars and refined grains, the need for higher protein levels, and snack and meal preparation strategies that can mitigate hunger. Not to be overlooked, the revised DASH diet continues to recommend consuming zero to minimal sodium.

Sodium Decrease

As a result, adhering to the DASH diet's permitted foods and recommended portion sizes will automatically reduce your sodium intake. In addition to the naturally reduced sodium content of the DASH diet, however, you can further reduce your sodium intake by doing any of the following:

Salt-free cookery of hot cereal, pasta, and rice;

As an alternative to adding salt to cuisine, using salt-free flavorings or spices.

Selecting foods labeled "low sodium", "sodium-free", or "no salt added"; and

When consuming tinned foods, thoroughly rinse them to reduce their sodium content.

I'll be honest with you: low-sodium drinks and foods can taste a touch bland compared to the majority of high-sodium and salt-containing foods. If you find that going cold turkey on high-sodium foods is too difficult, begin by reducing your intake gradually. Increase the amount of low-sodium foods you consume daily and reduce the amount of salt you consume until you reach the maximum daily recommended amounts of sodium, which are less than 2,6 00 milligrams if you are not hypertensive and less than 2 ,10 00 milligrams if you are already hypertensive. Slow and steady prevails, so the saying goes.

On Your Mark, Get Set, DASH!

Now is when you'll have to put your money where your mouth is, and you'll be putting into practice the fundamental principles and ideas underlying the DASH diet that you've learned so far.

Ultimately, a diet is not something to be read, but rather something to be implemented. Here is some useful advice to help you get off to a good start:

Baby Steps: Rome wasn't built in a day, so don't expect to transition fully and joyfully to the DASH diet overnight. It's like asking a smoker to quit cold turkey or a narcissist to stop talking about themselves immediately.

Going too quickly with something that will radically alter your way of life increases your risk of failure, and by a large margin. Focus by tackling it step-by-step, day-by-day, week-by-week, and month-by-month. For instance, you can progressively increase your vegetable and fruit consumption from one serving per day to two servings on the first week, then one serving per week until you reach four to five servings per day, while simultaneously reducing your consumption of meat and processed foods. Alternately, you could replace 2 or 2 of your daily servings of refined grains with whole grains during the first wcck, and then gradually increase the daily servings of whole grains while decreasing the daily servings of refined grains by 2 serving per week until you have completely replaced refined grains with whole grains.

Forgive And Reward: Remember that switching to the DASH diet can be difficult, particularly if you've been consuming high-sodium treats for years. Consequently, you are destined to make mistakes occasionally. The key to successfully transitioning to and maintaining the complete DASH diet is learning to forgive yourself. Everyone makes errors, so why should you be an exception? Simply acknowledge that you've made a mistake, learn from it, and make every effort to avoid the same situation or factors in the future.

It is also essential to give yourself something to anticipate. As a result, you should reward yourself with some of your favored treats once a week - in moderation, of course - to maintain your motivation on the DASH diet. Without a powerful motivation, such as your favored food, you will feel deprived and will simply be working. This increases the likelihood that you will become discouraged or lose interest in maintaining the diet for optimal health.

Regular physical activity performed at the appropriate intensity will be extremely beneficial for lowering blood pressure. Combining the DASH diet with regular, low-intensity exercises such as 6 0-minute neighborhood walks can reduce blood pressure significantly more than dieting alone.

If you find it difficult to adhere to difficult tasks, such as nutrition, you will need the assistance of others. Create an informal team that can assist you in adopting the DASH diet and stopping hypertension. Your team should consist of your doctor for medical oversight and close family and friends for moral and logistical support.

Not An Extreme

Healthy living in general and healthy nutrition in particular do not require an extreme lifestyle. The key is to consume the appropriate foods in sufficient quantities so that, on average, you consume significantly more healthy foods than harmful ones. However, it is acceptable to consume some of your favorite high-sodium foods occasionally and in small or moderate quantities. Therefore, moderation is essential.

Now is the time to hit the ground running by preparing 9 deliciously healthy dishes for the DASH diet in order to reduce blood pressure!

According to the World Health Organization (WHO), elevated blood pressure is one of the most prevalent chronic conditions worldwide. An estimated 76 million Americans suffer from hypertension/high blood pressure. This indicates that they experience a consistent increase in arterial pressure. Consequently, the heart must labor harder. A sustained increase in blood pressure may also result in a stroke or heart attack. In addition, as time passes, the arteries become less elastic and scarred, which causes the heart muscle to become weaker, denser, and less effective at pumping blood. In addition, the arteries are unable to deliver sufficient blood to the organs for their appropriate function, affecting the organs. Eating a nutritious diet and decreasing your sodium intake are essential for reducing your risk of developing high blood pressure. This is the premise upon which the DASH diet is based. Dietary Approaches to Stop Hypertension is what DASH stands for. The National Institutes of Health funded the original research that led to the development of this regimen, which was created by medical and nutritional scientists. This indicates that the DASH diet is not just another diet fad designed to promote products and generate profits. DASH is not a fad diet, but rather a realistic dietary plan that encourages permanent lifestyle changes.

The DASH diet is described

The DASH diet is a well-thought-out eating plan that is balanced, adaptable, and designed to aid in the development of a lifelong heart-healthy diet. This plan emphasizes limiting cholesterol and saturated fat as part of your daily and weekly nutritional objectives, rather than focusing on special foods. This diet emphasizes the importance of consuming more foods rich in nutrients that lower blood pressure, particularly minerals (magnesium, calcium, and potassium), fiber, and protein. It comprises foods considered to be nutritional powerhouses in order to meet the Institute of Medicine's nutritional recommendations. When following this diet, you will consume a greater quantity of vegetables, whole cereals, and fruits than you would on a normal diet.

The DASH diet recommends organizing your meals around fruits, vegetables, and grains and limiting your consumption of high-saturated-fat foods such as fatty meats, full-fat dairy, and tropical oils such as palm oil, palm kernel oil, and coconut oil. You must also limit your consumption of candies and sugar-sweetened beverages. Consequently, your diet and menu will include fish, legumes, low-fat dairy products, poultry, nuts, and vegetable oils. Regardless of your dietary preferences, the DASH diet is easy to follow.

Caution is advised before undertaking DASH. Several adverse effects are associated with this diet. High fiber consumption is likely to result in diarrhea and bloating, according to experts. To prevent these side effects, you should progressively increase your consumption of whole grains, vegetables, and fruits.

Who Developed the DASH eating plan?

A group of fifty researchers, comprised of dietitians and physicians from prestigious medical institutions such as

Duke University School of Medicine, Johns Hopkins Medical Center, and Harvard Medical Center, set out to devise a diet that would aid in lowering blood pressure. Volunteers who participated in a study experienced a reduction in blood pressure and weight loss, although the latter was not the primary objective of the study. Over the years, the DASH diet plan has been and continues to be widely regarded as an effective method for lowering blood pressure and effortlessly losing weight. In fact, for the eighth consecutive year, U.S. News and World Report has ranked this diet as the Best Overall Diet out of forty other diets.

Who Should adhere to the DASH Diet?

This regimen was designed for those with high blood pressure or who have been advised to lower their blood pressure by their general practitioner, who have cardiovascular disease or are at risk of developing cardiovascular disease. You can also follow this regimen if you have hypertension symptoms such as fatigue, chest pain, and headaches. However, there are no restrictions on who can follow the DASH diet, as it promotes a healthful lifestyle in addition to lowering blood pressure.

Reasons to Choose the DASH Diet

It is far superior to take medication to manage hypertension and prehypertension symptoms than to watch what you consume. Here are some of the benefits of choosing the DASH diet:

The DASH diet is accommodating. The premise upon which this diet is based allows it to be combined with any other diet, as it is compatible with other lifestyles and cultures. Furthermore, it is not restrictive, so it can be modified to accommodate dietary restrictions such as vegan and vegetarian diets. It is also adaptable to gluten-free, halal, and kosher diets. What else is there? This diet is appropriate for both infants and adults.

The DASH regimen is cost-free. You are not required to pay a subscription fee or purchase any products to begin the DASH diet. You only need to maintain your regular food expenditure; however, your grocery store food selections will shift to emphasize more nutrient-dense foods. This also applies when dining in establishments, as you should prioritize healthy beverages. The recommended foods in this diet plan are simple but varied, ensuring that you will have a variety of foods on your table.

The DASH eating plan eradicates metabolic syndrome. The DASH diet can eliminate metabolic syndrome regardless of whether you are aware you have it or not. If you have three or more of the following health conditions, you have a metabolic condition: high blood pressure, high triglyceride levels, low

HDL cholesterol levels, high blood sugar, or a large waist circumference.

Who does the Dash Diet cater to?

The DASH diet was created to assist individuals with prehypertension and hypertension. The evidence suggests that lifestyle adjustments combined with the DASH diet will regulate blood pressure more effectively than medication. This diet emphasizes ingesting as little sodium as possible, giving you an advantage against blood pressure issues. This makes it an excellent choice for individuals with a history of cardiovascular disease and those who are at risk for or presently managing type 2 diabetes.

Types of DASH Diet

You can choose between two forms of the DASH diet, depending on your individual health requirements.

The DASH reduced sodium diet. This variant of the DASH diet is based on a daily sodium intake limit of 2,10 00 mg.

The conventional DASH diet. This option limits your daily sodium intake to 2,6 00 milligrams.

Chapter 4: How Effective Is The Dash Diet?

Dash diet is not a "diet" in the traditional sense; rather, it is a program based on solid and well-researched nutritional facts, designed to assist you in developing a diet that will decrease your sodium intake, thereby lowering your blood pressure through the food you eat. DASH aims to assist and guide individuals in making well-informed dietary and lifestyle decisions that will result in substantial and long-lasting health benefits.

It is a fact that elevated blood pressure, also known as hypertension, can be a potentially fatal condition. It can progress to a variety of life-threatening conditions, including coronary artery disease, stroke, and heart failure.

Despite this, a significant portion of the population, approximately 6 6 % of both sexes, still suffers from hypertension, and many of them remain undiagnosed. There is a high likelihood that either you or someone you know has hypertension.

The DASH diet focuses primarily on reducing sodium intake, one of the leading causes of hypertension today. The majority of individuals are unaware of how much salt they consume on a daily basis solely by consuming "normal" foods. The recommended daily salt intake is approximately 2,6 00 milligrams, whereas the dash diet aims to reduce this to approximately 2 ,10 00 mg.

Compare these figures to the 2 ,2 90 mg of sodium found in the average quarter-pound cheeseburger. That is nearly half of an individual's daily allowance in a single burger, and even more if you follow the DASH Diet. This comparison demonstrates how simple it is for people to consume significantly more salt than the daily recommendation without realizing it. Even for those who already consume what they believe to be a healthy and balanced diet consisting of plenty of salads and healthy food options, there is a risk that their salt consumption is much higher than they realize. The high sodium content of condiments and salad dressings suggests that your salad may not be as healthful as you believe.

Here are some of the most important dietary modifications suggested by the DASH Diet:

Replace treats and desserts with an abundance of fresh produce.

Selecting foods high in fiber over those high in refined carbohydrates.

Replacing whole milk products with alternatives that are minimal in fat or fat-free.

Substituting water and club soda for sugary soft beverages.

It is essential to keep in mind that the DASH Diet is about more than just healthful eating. The DASH Diet is a lifestyle philosophy that promotes health. This requires more than just dietary adjustments. Below is a list of additional areas of your life where modifications may be necessary:

Attempt to engage in at least 6 0 minutes of daily physical activity.

If you are attempting to lose weight, you should set short-term, attainable goals for your weight loss. It is much more motivating to achieve a series of small goals than it is to strive for a single massive goal in the distant future.

If you have been diagnosed with hypertension and are taking prescription medication for it, you should continue to take your medication and maintain regular doctor's appointments to monitor your progress.

The DASH Diet is an approach to weight reduction and healthy living based on common sense. It is not surprising that it has garnered a great deal of interest and is gaining popularity rapidly. There are benefits to following the DASH Diet even for those who perceive themselves to be healthy. Maintaining a high-fibre, low-fat, and low-sodium diet, along with regular exercise, will facilitate weight loss and ensure that it is maintained. In some instances, altering this routine could save someone's life.

What exactly are Smoothies?

In the United Kingdom, nutritionists recommend consuming five portions of fruits and vegetables per day. The majority of us comprehend the benefits of a well-balanced, fruit- and vegetable-rich diet. However, it is not always simple to convey this message to our offspring. Generally, a child's dietary habits will be determined by their parents, but it is common for them to require smoothies for additional energy throughout the day. Rarely will they include fruits and vegetables in their decision-making process for smoothies.

Generally speaking, children appreciate drinking fruit juices. The issue is, however, that even fresh, homemade juice, which is unquestionably healthier than sweets or chips, lacks certain essential nutrients. The straightforward act of extracting juice from a fruit eliminates both soluble and insoluble fiber, which we require. These are essential for the health and upkeep of our digestive system.

Most people have a fundamental understanding of fibre and are aware that it is an essential component of a healthy diet. However, the fact that there are both soluble and insoluble fibers will be news to the majority.

We are most knowledgeable about insoluble fiber. It regulates our digestive function, ensuring proper bowel function and preventing constipation and its associated complications, such as hemorrhoids (piles). Most people will be unfamiliar with soluble fibre, despite its importance to our general health and wellbeing. It has been shown to assist in lowering cholesterol and regulating blood sugar levels, as well as preventing more serious conditions such as colon cancer.

It is common for individuals to experience what could be termed an afternoon "slump" This represents a decline in vitality levels. During such situations, it is tempting to reach for the cookie jar or the chocolate shelf in the pantry. This is the ideal opportunity to prepare a nutritious smoothie. It is essential to introduce children to smoothies at a young age in order to firmly establish this option in their minds and encourage the development of healthy food habits that will serve them well in the future.

Chapter 5: Hypertension Today

Many of us are aware that hypertension, also known as elevated blood pressure, is a serious medical condition. We are aware that prolonged, uncontrolled hypertension can have a variety of negative effects on our health. However, when do blood pressure levels become abnormal? What blood pressure readings must be taken at the doctor's office for someone to be diagnosed with excessive blood pressure? Let's examine the numbers and their significance.

How is excessive blood pressure defined?

When your blood pressure is measured, you will see two numbers, such as 2 20/80 (read as "2 20 over 80"). The first number represents the systolic pressure, or the pressure in the arteries when the heart contracts. Diastolic pressure, on the other hand, is the lowest pressure in your blood vessels as your heart relaxes between pulses.

These two numbers indicate to your physician whether or not your blood pressure is healthful. Any systolic blood pressure reading over 2 6 0 or diastolic reading over 80 is considered excessive blood pressure. Obviously, healthy numbers will differ based on a person's age and health, such as for a child, an adult, or a pregnant woman.

The relationship between children and elevated blood pressure

From infancy to adolescence, hypertension is less prevalent in children, but it is still conceivable. In contrast to adults, there will be appropriate weight ranges for children based on their gender, height, and age. These are determined based on the blood pressure readings of healthy adolescents. You should consult your physician regarding your child's blood pressure reading based on their gender, age, and weight percentile.

High blood pressure during pregnancy

Pregnant women may experience high blood pressure. Readings above 2 8 0 systolic or 90 diastolic are considered high. Normal blood pressure readings during pregnancy should be below 2 20 systolic and 80 diastolic. However, hypertension is more prevalent during pregnancy, with 8% of pregnant women developing some form of the condition.

There are two types of hypertension that can develop during pregnancy. These consist of:

Chronic hypertension occurs when a woman's blood pressure is excessive even before she becomes pregnant or if her blood pressure rises before 20 weeks of pregnancy.

After 20 weeks of pregnancy, high blood pressure issues manifest as hypertensive disorders of pregnancy. The majority of them will vanish once the mother gives birth.

Chapter 6: The Dash Diet Was Superior To The Western And Mediterranean Diets For Depression

Cherian and her colleagues investigated whether diet could be used to reduce the risk of depression for their study. They utilized data from the Memory and Aging Project at Rush University, which tracks the aging of non-dementia-afflicted senior Americans, to investigate the onset of the condition and factors that may influence dementia.

The investigation followed 968 individuals with an average age of 82 for more than six years. The participants were monitored for depressive symptoms and complete food intake questionnaires. The researchers classified the participants into groups based on how closely they adhered to the DASH diet, the Mediterranean diet, the MIND diet, or the traditional Western diet, as determined by the food-intake questionnaires.

The Mediterranean diet consists of plant-based foods, the substitution of butter with olive or canola oil, the restriction of red meat consumption, and the consumption of fish and poultry. The MIND Diet (Mediterranean-DASH Intervention for Neurodegenerative Delay) is a hybrid of the DASH and Mediterranean diets that emphasizes nutrients believed to promote brain health, such as leafy green vegetables, nuts, berries, olive oil, and a low- to moderate-alcohol consumption.

According to Cherian, the traditional Western diet is traditionally higher in red meat, sodium, and saturated fats, such as butter, and lower in fruits and vegetables. It contains more refined and processed foods, including white bread, nibble foods, and sugar."

According to the study, those who followed the DASH diet had the lowest risk of developing depression, whereas those who followed the traditional Western diet had the highest risk.

The study only establishes a correlation between the DASH diet and a reduced incidence of depression; it does not demonstrate that the diet causes this effect. Cherian notes, however, that the researchers attempted to isolate the effect of diet by controlling for other factors that may contribute to the development of depression.

What exactly is the DASH diet? A Guide to the Plan for Weight Loss and Blood Pressure Reduction

Your DASH Diet Primer

Dietary Approaches to Stop Hypertension (DASH) is a balanced, varied eating plan that provides a practical nutrition solution to help you reach your objectives. All of the fad diets and nutritional trends in the world complicate healthy dining. We will disregard this and instead focus on a dietary style in which you can have complete confidence. Here, we will examine why the DASH diet is so distinct and superior to what you may be used to eating.

Chapter 7: How The Dash Diet Promotes Weight Loss And Reduces Blood Pressure

The DASH diet is notable for its abundance of fruits, vegetables, and low-fat dairy products, as well as its generally low saturated fat content. The DASH diet's blood pressure lowering properties are frequently attributed to its naturally high potassium, calcium, and magnesium content, which are found in abundance in the diet's wide variety of foods.

Without Sacrificing Flavor, Reduce Sodium Intake

The DASH diet promotes foods and dishes that are typically low in sodium without sacrificing flavor. However, novices may require some adjustment, particularly if they are accustomed to robust and savory flavors. Here are some tips to help you progressively reduce your sodium intake:

- Become familiar with sodium-free seasonings and flavors that can be used in place of salt.

- Rinse canned foods, if feasible, to remove a portion of the added sodium.

- When preparing cereal, pasta, or rice, refrain from adding salt or other sodium-containing seasonings.

Choose foods with labels such as "very low sodium", "low sodium", "sodium-free", or "no salt added" when shopping in supermarkets.

If you make it a habit to read food labels, you may be startled to learn that certain foods, such as some canned soups, instant cereals, canned vegetables, and even apparently innocent deli-sliced turkey, contain extremely high levels of sodium.

There is a perceptible distinction between regular and low-sodium foods. To give your taste buds time to adjust, reduce the amount of table salt you use and progressively incorporate lower sodium options into your diet. There are also herb spice blends and other salt-free seasonings that can aid in the transition.

Starting Strong

Beginning any type of regimen can be difficult, particularly at first. This is one of the most common reasons why people resign. The key to achieving success with the DASH diet is to acclimate into your new eating habits. Here are some suggestions to assist you in doing so:

- Permit yourself time to adapt. Give yourself time to acclimate if you dislike vegetables and fruits or if you need to drastically reduce your intake of sweet treats. Add or remove one serving per day from each food group in infant steps. While making changes to your diet, make a note of any positive or negative changes in your body, so you can pinpoint your problem areas (for example, you observe you have more gas after eating vegetables or beans, or you experience diarrhea after consuming grains). By identifying your problem areas, you will be able to consult with medical professionals.

- Include manageable physical activities in your routine. Increasing your physical activity in order to lower your blood pressure is a fantastic method to improve the efficacy of the DASH diet. If your schedule allows you to exercise or visit the gym, you should do so. Alternatively, you can increase your physical activity by walking or ascending the stairs more frequently. Do not attempt to accomplish more than you are capable of or your time permits.

- Recognize your accomplishments and allow for occasional lapses. Reward your achievements with non-food treats, such as going to a movie or buying new clothes (which may be a good idea, given that you will undoubtedly lose weight). Do not punish yourself if you make a mistake. Remember that changing behaviors is a lengthy process. You can determine what caused the setback and then continue from where you left off.

- Do not be reluctant to seek assistance. If you find it challenging to adhere to the DASH diet, seek assistance. Share your concerns with your dietitian or reach out to the DASH diet community for assistance.

Intake of Calories on the DASH Diet

The DASH dietary guidelines emphasize the consumption of a wide variety of food groups in varying quantities based on an individual's characteristics. These dietary groups and their recommended serving sizes are determined by a person's age, gender, and level of physical activity. Before determining your own DASH diet guidelines, you must estimate your calorie requirements. The first two tables will assist you in estimating your daily caloric requirements. Consider your physical activity in order to determine your estimated daily calorie intake. Sedentary is defined as little to no physical activity, moderately active as walking 2 .10 to 6 miles per day in addition to mild physical activity, and active as exercising at the intensity recommended by the 28-day plan that follows.

2 . What is DASH Diet?

In recent years, the Dash Diet has gained popularity due to its ability to lower blood pressure and reduce the body's susceptibility to a variety of diseases. Dietary Approaches to Stop Hypertension, or DASH, is a program that was created and initially disseminated to patients who wished to reduce their sodium intake.

Since the Dash Diet is based on the premise that reducing sodium consumption will result in a natural reduction in blood pressure, it follows that this eating plan is ideal for those who are working to improve their health and eliminate hypertension. Those who were assigned to follow the Dash Diet, however, reported that their efforts to reduce body fat were fruitful. As a result, people all over the world began following the Dash Diet.

In the 2 990s, when the Dash Diet was initially developed, its primary dietary categories consisted of starchy foods and grains. It gradually evolved into the form we recognize today, which emphasizes consuming a broad variety of fresh fruits and vegetables, low-fat dairy products, and nutrient-dense protein sources such as seeds, beans, and nuts. Healthy whole grains, such as bread prepared with whole wheat, can be included in the diet, but only in small amounts.

Empty carbs, such as those found in processed white bread and other foods, should be eliminated from the diet because they raise blood pressure and increase the total number of calories ingested. Dieters who are dedicated to the Dash eating plan and strictly adhere to it report that it is one of the most effective strategies for weight loss and overall body improvement.

Organizing meals for breakfast, lunch, and dinner is quite uncomplicated. The cuisine includes low-fat dairy products such as milk and yogurt, an abundance of fresh fruit, leafy greens such as spinach and vegetables such as broccoli, lean meats such as chicken or salmon, and a protein-rich dish of beans.

In order to facilitate successful weight loss, the Dash Diet is typically divided into two phases: The first phase lasts two weeks and concentrates on reducing abdominal obesity. It is the longest phase and is said to be the one that dieters remain on for the remainder of their lives. Dieters are permitted to ingest a wider variety of foods during this phase compared to the first two weeks of the diet.

It makes no difference why someone decides to begin the Dash Diet; the fact is that adhering to this regimen results in a healthier body overall, and these benefits cannot be disputed.

Why Dash Diet?

Because there are so many different diets to choose from, it can be difficult to determine which one is best adapted to your body and lifestyle. Thankfully, there are a few that tend to work on a broad scale for individuals, despite the fact that their goals may vary slightly. For instance, the Dash Diet is a nutritional regimen initially designed for individuals diagnosed with hypertension, another term for elevated blood pressure. Dash was created because doctors and dietitians observed that patients' blood pressure increased when they consumed sodium. In response to this finding, Dash was created so that patients could be placed on a diet containing less sodium.

Patients who followed the Dash Diet, on the other hand, reported both weight loss and a reduction in blood pressure as a result of the diet. Since then, the ketogenic diet has become one of the most well-known diets to emerge since the 2 990s. Those who incorporate the Dash Diet into their daily lives can benefit from its adaptability, which is another compelling argument in its favor. Individuals who wish to reduce their sodium intake in an uncomplicated fashion have the option of selecting the standard level of sodium consumption, which is 2,6 00 milligrams. The recommended daily intake of sodium is reduced to 2 ,10 00 mg for individuals who have expressed a desire to significantly reduce their sodium consumption. This again affords some flexibility in the situation.

A number of diets are regarded as being extremely restrictive, but the Dash Diet is not one of them. The fact that this diet can be concluded in two phases is one of its numerous advantageous features. During the first phase of the diet, which lasts approximately two weeks, the dieter should avoid sugary and carbohydrate foods as much as possible. This is done to ensure that the maximum amount of abdominal fat is lost in the first two weeks of the regimen. During the second phase of the program, nutrient-dense carbohydrates are progressively reintroduced to the diet, with the expectation that the body will have the increased metabolism required to process them. Dieters should continue to adhere as closely as possible to Phase Two of the diet in order to maintain their weight loss over the long term.

A further benefit of this diet is that Phase Two is so readily adaptable to individuals' current eating habits. This is accomplished through simple substitutions, such as transitioning from refined to whole grains and snacking on protein-rich foods. After all is said and done, there is relatively little sacrifice but a substantial gain.

How It Operates

Dietary Approaches to Stop Hypertension (DASH) suggests consuming fruits, vegetables, low-fat milk, whole grains, fish, poultry, beans, and nuts. It recommends reducing consumption of red meat, foods and beverages with added carbohydrates, and sodium. This diet is heart-healthy because it reduces your consumption of saturated and trans fats while increasing your consumption of potassium, magnesium, calcium, and protein. All of these nutrients are believed to contribute to blood pressure regulation.

The diet involves ingesting a specific number of servings of each of the recommended foods (see list above). The National Heart, Lung, and Blood Institute (NHLBI) has provided sample meal plans based on daily caloric intakes of 2 ,600, 2,000, and 2,600 calories. This equates to approximately 6-8 servings of grains or grain products (whole grains are recommended), 8 -10 servings of vegetables, 8 -10 servings of fruits, 2-6 servings of low fat dairy foods, 2 or fewer 6 -ounce portions of meat, poultry, or fish, 2-6 servings of fats and oils, and 8 -10 servings of nuts, seeds, or dry beans per week for a 2000-calorie diet. Whole grains are advised. It is recommended that you consume no more than five servings of sweets and added carbohydrates per week. The plan specifies the correct portion sizes for each of these food groups.

Consuming fewer carbohydrates and more protein or unsaturated fats may also be beneficial to one's cardiac health. The clinical trial known as OmniHeart (Optimal Macronutrient Intake Trial to Prevent Heart Disease) found that replacing approximately 2 0% of the calories from carbohydrates with protein (particularly plant proteins like legumes, nuts, and seeds) or monounsaturated fats (olive oil, canola oil, nuts) decreased blood pressure, LDL cholesterol, and triglycerides in individuals with early or stage 2 hypertension.

Particularly, the substitution of carbohydrates with unsaturated lipids contributed to an increase in "good" HDL cholesterol. The effect was not solely the result of consuming additional fats and proteins; rather, it was the result of exchanging one caloric source for another in such a manner that the total number of calories consumed remained roughly the same. In order to consume 2000 calories per day, you should consume approximately 8 to 10 servings of whole cereals, 10 servings of vegetables, 2 to 6 servings of fruits, 2 servings of low-fat dairy foods, one 6 - ounce serving of fish, poultry, or meat, and 2 to 6 servings of unsaturated fats. Additionally, you should consume 7-8 servings per week of legumes, nuts, or seeds.

To adhere to the plan, one must first determine their intended caloric intake and then divide the recommended number of servings from each food group into smaller portions throughout the day. Therefore, it is necessary to plan your meals in advance. The handbook provided by the NHLBI contains a sample diet for one day that adheres to a salt restriction of either 26 00 mg or 2 10 00 mg, as well as a week's worth of recipes. There are numerous suggestions on how to incorporate DASH foods and reduce sodium intake. Additionally, the NHLBI maintains a database of "heart healthy" recipes accessible online.

Chicken Quesadillas

Ingredients

2 cup onions, minced
 8 oz boneless, skinless chicken breasts

 12 whole wheat tortillas 8 inches in
diameter

1 cup salsa
2 cup tomatoes, minced
2 cup cilantro, minced

Preparation

1. Each chicken breast should be
   chopped into bite-sized pieces.

2.

3. In a nonstick skillet, heat the chicken and onions until they are well cooked. Turn off heat and stir in salsa, cilantro, tomatoes, and chili.

4.

5. Use a platter to assemble the tortillas. Spread 1 cup chicken mixture on one side of the tortilla.

6.

7. Leave 1 inch around the edge. Sprinkle with cheese, then fold in half.

8.

9. Place the chicken quesadillas on a baking sheet lined with parchment paper.

10.

11. Lightly coat the quesadillas with vegetable oil. Bake for up to ten mins or until they turn light brown.

12.

You can cut in half, or just eat as-is.

Cups Of Cherry-Chicken Lettuce

Ingredients

Vegetable oil cooking spray
4 teaspoon olive oil
4 tablespoons rice vinegar
4 tablespoons of low-sodium teriyaki sauce

8 green onions, minced 8 small lettuce leaves pieces

1/2   pound cubed, boneless, skinless chicken breast
1/2   cup chopped almonds
1/2   teaspoon iodized salt
1/2   teaspoon ground black pepper
2 teaspoon ground ginger 2 1 cups carrots, shredded

2 cups sweet cherries, pitted and
coarsely chopped
 2 tablespoon raw honey

Preparation

1. Season the chicken with salt & pepper
    Heat a nonstick skillet by coating it
    with vegetable oil cooking spray.
2. over   medium   heat.

3. To cook chicken cubes, heat until
    golden   brown.

4. After removing the chicken from the
    heat, stir in the carrots, greenonions
    and   almonds.

5. Mix the honey, vinegar, and teriyaki
    sauce in a bowl.

6. Pour onto the chicken cubes to coat. Divide the seasoned chicken cubes between the lettuce leaves and fold over to make a cup.

7. Serve immediately on a plate.

Chapter 8: Whole Grains And Carbohydrate-Rich Produce

Let's face it: nearly everyone enjoys carbohydrate-rich foods, and although very-low-carb diets may help some individuals lose weight in the short term, they are not particularly sustainable and are certainly not very delightful. The DASH diet does not recommend avoiding carbohydrates; rather, it recommends consuming the most fiber- and nutrient-dense versions. This is a message I can undoubtedly support. Brown rice, quinoa, whole-grain bread, whole-grain pasta, and potatoes (of any variety) are DASH-compliant.

Size of each serving: 12 slices of whole-grain bread, 0.21 cup of brown rice or quinoa, and 12 medium-sized potatoes or sweet potatoes.

VEGETABLES

Vegetables are, simply stated, the most essential component of any diet. The high potassium content of the majority of vegetables, particularly leafy greens, plays a crucial role in blood pressure regulation. By regulating the fluid balance in your body, your kidneys play an important role in blood pressure management. The sodium and potassium you consume further affect this equilibrium. The majority of people consume far more sodium than potassium, which hinders the kidneys' ability to regulate blood pressure effectively. The majority of individuals can restore this balance by increasing their potassium intake and decreasing their sodium intake. Vegetables contain an abundance of other beneficial nutrients and antioxidant compounds. Vegetables' high fiber content promotes satiety and may prevent weight gain from a weight management perspective. A study published in The Journal of Nutrition in 2009 found that women who increased their fiber intake over time gained less weight and body fat. Only about half of the population meets the American Heart Association's daily fiber intake recommendation of 36.0 grams per day.

Size of one serving: 121 cup cooked vegetables, such as broccoli or Brussels sprouts, and 12 cups fresh vegetables, such as spinach.

FRUIT

Occasionally, popular "diets" recommend eliminating Fruit because it contains a moderate quantity of natural sugars. If you've heard this, I urge you to disregard it and embrace fruit as a very healthful component of the DASH diet and a vital component of long life and good health. Fruit, in addition to being delectable, is abundant in potassium, fiber, and other essential nutrients that support blood pressure and weight management.

12 pieces of fruit of medium size, such as an apple or banana, and 0.21 cup of fruit, such as raspberries or strawberries, constitute one serving.

Milk Alternatives And Low-Fat Milk Products

Low-Fat Dairy And Replacements

The DASH dietary plan includes dairy products and alternatives for a number of reasons. The high calcium content of these foods is believed to play a significant role in blood pressure regulation because it modifies the hormones responsible for blood vessel tension. The high protein content promotes weight management and weight loss because protein not only makes us feel satisfied, but also requires additional energy for our bodies to break it down. This primarily explains why studies, such as a 2012 510-review published in The American Journal of Clinical Nutrition, tend to find that adequate protein intake is typically associated with improved outcomes in terms of weight management and appetite control.

Chapter 9: Strategies And Tactics And Planning

When beginning the DASH diet, you'll also need to understand your metabolism so that you can determine how much food you should consume. In addition to motivation, you must be able to eliminate unhealthy foods from your home before beginning. If you eliminate savory temptation, you are less likely to consume it. Try to gain your family's support, as it will benefit their health and well-being as well. A positive and motivating environment can determine whether or not you will adhere to a diet over the long term.

Tips

Here are several suggestions that will facilitate your transition to the DASH methodology:

Always opt for whole grain options. This is applicable to bread and pasta due to their significantly higher fiber content and other nutrient benefits. This also holds true for selecting brown rice over white rice.

-Dried beans contain less sodium than canned beans, even after rinsing the canned beans.

-Limit your condiments. Numerous condiments and dressings are loaded with sodium and sugar. When you combine these, you may not even realize how much you are consuming. A tablespoon of most condiments is sufficient for flavoring, while a pinch of seasoning is sufficient.

-It may take a week or more for your taste buds to acclimate to the new seasonings. Instead of becoming agitated because you believe you cannot do it, adhere to the diet. Within two weeks, your taste buds will typically adjust and you will have diminished cravings for the eliminated foods. Alternately, begin substituting them with comparable foods that adhere to the diet. For instance, substitute dessert with fruit, which is still delicious but more nutritious.

-Whenever possible, use fresh herbs and seasonings rather than dried ones, as this will intensify the flavor of your food. The majority of dried seasonings pale in comparison to their fresh counterparts.

-Eliminating extra calories from beverages is an essential strategy for reducing sugar intake. As much as feasible, switch to water or herbal tea to improve your hydration. Approximately 70% of American adults are chronically dehydrated because the majority of liquids they consume contain sodium, a diuretic. By substituting water for juice, soda, and sugar in coffee, you can eliminate between 36,000 and 500,000 calories per day. Add a slice of lemon, lime, or citrus to your water if you find it difficult to drink it plain.

-Try to maintain your resolve when presented foods you cannot consume. Remember the reason for your commitment.

If you are aware of when you are likely to deviate from your diet, attempt to plan accordingly. If you know you'll be compelled to stop for fast food on the way home, keep a healthy DASH-friendly snack in the car so you won't need or want to stop.

-If you're unfamiliar with portion sizes, begin pre-portioning your food so you know you're staying within your limits. Using a calorie or diet program is also a good idea so that you can keep a food journal and comprehend how much you eat daily.

Try to drink at least eight 8-ounce portions of water per day. Hydration is essential for good health, and you'll need it to eliminate sodium from your body and maintain hydration after exercise. Consider that you may require more than 8 glasses (648 oz) of water per day, depending on your weight, the conditions, and your level of activity.

-Try to concentrate on your diet. Are you snacking because you're bored or because you're genuinely hungry? Frequently, we do not realize why we are reaching for food. Frequently, we can even confuse thirst for hunger. If you sense the urge to snack, drink a glass of water first to see if it goes away.

DASH Weight-loss

When using DASH to achieve weight loss goals, it is essential to comprehend how weight loss occurs. Your body operates on a simple equation of calories in versus calories out. Consume too many calories and you will gain weight; consume too few and you will lose weight. Depending on how much weight you need to lose, you'll need to operate with a deficit of 510 000 to 12 000 calories. Determine your BMR based on your age, gender, and level of activity, and calculate the amount of food you should consume to lose weight safely.

DASH Cooking Techniques

We've seen that frying is a huge no-no when it comes to DASH cooking, as it's simply too high in fat to suit the parameters. Nonstick cookware is also optimal for reducing the amount of fat in a meal, as it eliminates the need for fat to prevent food from sticking. If you're unfamiliar with cooking grains, a rice cooker is also an excellent option because it often doubles as a vegetable steamer. Roasting vegetables helps bring out their flavor, but not all vegetables are suitable for roasting. Similar to grilling, broiling allows excess fat to trickle away from the food and into a tray below. Rubs and seasonings that are lower in sodium and sugar than sauces can also be used. Both steaming and poaching are optimal methods for DASH cooking because no added fats are used. If you don't have a steamer, you can achieve a comparable effect by wrapping the food in aluminum foil and baking it in its own juice.

Two Week Plan

Now that you are familiar with the fundamentals of what and how to consume on the DASH diet, you will learn how to put it all together. These are two phase one sample schedules for the original DASH and the DASH for weight loss diets. The items marked with an asterisk (*) are included in the recipe segment that follows.

easily keeping

Chapter 10: Hurertenon Is An Alternative Term For High Blood Pressure.

SUSTOLIS BLOOD RRESSURE — The point at which arteriolar pressure is high (when the ventricles are in contraction). The initial measurement in a blood urea measurement. Government and health organizations continue to pressure the food industry to reduce the sodium content of processed foods. The New York City Health Department led the National The Salt Reduction Initiative in the United States and several other health-related organizations joined the effort. Their objective was to reduce the salinity in the United States by 20% by 2012 48. The solicitation was effective with food manufacturers and eateries that voluntarily agreed to reduce the amount of lead in their products. In addition, the U.S. Department of Health and Human Servces, along with a number of other federal and private sector organizations, spearheaded the Mllon Heart initiative. Between 2012 and 2012, their objective was to prevent one million heart attacks and strokes in the United States. Reduction of sodium levels in the diet to aid in lowering blood pressure was also a significant aspect of this initiative.

ASK YOUR DOCTOR THESE QUESTIONS

COULD THE DASH DIET HELP ME TO DECREASE MY BLOOD PRESSURE?

Can I follow the DASH diet if my blood pressure is already low? Will adhering to this diet permit me to discontinue taking blood pressure medication? There is some debate as to whether rats can adhere to the diet in the long run. The 20036 PREMIER Clnsal Tral (a multi-senter tral) examined the effect of diet on blood pressure and found that the results of the DASH diet were inferior to those of the original study. This difference was attributed to the fact that participants in the DASH study were given pre-prepared meals, whereas participants in the PREMIER study prepared their own meals. As a result, only half of the recommended fruit and vegetable servings were consumed in the PREMIER study, which negatively impacted the recommended daily allowances of potassium and magnesium. The researchers acknowledged that long-term success with the DASH diet was dubious, but they agreed that individuals should still be encouraged to adopt health interventions such as the DASH diet, as it does provide health benefits. In terms of heart health, the DASH diet was associated with a decline in high-density lipoprotein (HDL), the "good" cholesterol. Low HDL levels are regarded as a risk factor for coronary heart disease, whereas high HDL levels are believed to reduce the risk of heart disease. The decline was greatest in individuals who began with a high level of the harmful HDL cholesterol. Researchers agreed that the reasons for the decline in HDL levels required additional study, but conceded that the overall efficacy of the DASH diet in preventing heart disease was positive. While the long-term health effects of the DASH diet have yet to be established, the diet closely resembles the Mediterranean diet, which has been shown to have other health benefits, such as a reduced risk of heart disease and a lower blood pressure. The DASH diet is believed to provide comparable health advantages.

WHAT Is the dash board?

Dietary Arrroashe to Stor Hurertenon, or DASH, a diet resommened for reorles who want to rrevent or treat hypertension (also known as high blood pressure) and reduce their risk of cardiovascular disease. The DASH diet emphasizes fruits, veggies, whole grains, and lean meats. High blood pressure was much less common in people who followed a plant-based diet, specifically vegans and vegetarians. This is why the DASH diet emphasizes fruits and vegetables while also including lean sources of protein such as chicken, fish, and beans. It is low in red meat, salt, added sugar, and fat. Ssentt believe that one of the primary benefits of this diet is that it reduces salt intake. The standard DASH diet program recommends consuming no more than 12 teaspoons (2,360 milligrams) of sodium per day, which is consistent with the majority of national dietary guidelines. The reduced-sodium version is advised to contain no more than 36/48 teaspoons (12,510 mg) of salt per serving.

POTENTIAL BENEFITS

In addition to lowering blood pressure, the DASH diet offers a variety of additional benefits, such as weight loss and a reduced risk of cardiovascular disease. You should not expect DASH to help you lose weight on its own, as it was primarily designed to reduce blood pressure. Weght lo may be an additional hazard.

MAU AID WEIGHT LOSS

Whether or not you lose weight while following the DASH diet, your blood pressure will decrease. Nonetheless, if you already have high blood pressure, it is likely that you have been advised to lose weight. This is because your blood pressure is likely to be higher the heavier you are. In addition, it has been demonstrated that long weight reduces blood pressure. On the DASH diet, there is evidence that reorle can lose weight. Those who have lost weight on the DASH diet, however, have been on a calorie deficit, which means they have been instructed to consume fewer calories than they expend. Given that the DASH diet eliminates a significant amount of high-fat and high-sugar foods, individuals may discover that they automatically reduce their caloric intake and lose weight. Other roles may be required to retrace their steps. Either way, if you want to lose weight on the DASH diet, you'll still need to eat fewer calories.

Chapter 11: The Best Lifestyle Changes That Lower Blood Pressure Are: Reducing Sodium Intake

The most effective method to lower blood pressure and improve heart health may be to consume less salt. It may take up to two weeks for your taste buds to acclimate to a low-sodium diet.

One teaspoon of salt contains about 236,000 milligrams of sodium.

Eliminating table salt (which contains approximately 48.0% sodium) is an effective method to reduce sodium intake. However, the majority of sodium consumed originates from packaged and processed foods. Because sodium is present in all foods, it is vital to peruse the nutrition labels.

From frozen meals and chilled cuts to flatbread mixes and vegetable juices.

Other high-sodium foods include stews, broths, pasta in a can, sauces, and condiments. Choose low-sodium alternatives to packaged foods to reduce your sodium consumption. Substitute botanicals for salt.

TIP: The restaurant's cuisine may also be very high in sodium. Therefore, you should select nutritious food choices.

- Move

Regular physical activity can help manage blood pressure if you are physically strong enough to exercise. Additionally, it can help you lose weight, strengthen your heart, and alleviate tension.

The majority of adults should strive for at least five days per week of at least 360 minutes of exercise. However, it is not necessary to exercise for three hours at a time. Taking three 12-minute vigorous walks per day is also acceptable. Choose how to divide your weekly physical activity. Use the time you have to exercise if you have five minutes to spare.

Before beginning a new exercise regimen, consult with your physician to determine the best form of exercise for you.

• Aerobic exercise, such as cycling, swimming, stair climbing, rowing, brisk strolling, or running; • Strength training, such as weight lifting, squatting, or deadlifting

• Flexibility and stretching exercises or • Strength training exercises (at least twice per week)

Reduce your levels of tension

Work, relationships, finances, life changes, and emotional concerns are all sources of stress. While researchers continue to investigate the link between chronic stress and high blood pressure, eating unhealthy foods, avoiding physical activity, consuming too much alcohol, and smoking can increase blood pressure in response to stress.

The ability to cope with stress in a healthier manner will help reduce blood pressure. While you may not be able to eliminate all of your stress, there are measures you can take to maintain control:

• Do not overextend yourself. Set priorities and give yourself ample time to complete tasks.

• Learn to refuse. Even if others rely on you, you are not required to solve their problems.

• Speak it aloud. If you are experiencing issues at work, you should discuss the matter with your superior. Instead of arguing about a problem at home before going to bed, resolve it.

Take sufficient time to unwind. Take 12 510 or 20 minutes per day to sit quietly and disconnect from technology.

• Devote time to a friend. Invest in cultivating encouraging and supportive relationships.

• Do something you like. Whether you prefer tinkering in the kitchen or the garage, enjoy yourself and release the tension in your body.

I would like to recommend the following advice if your stress becomes unmanageable and you are seeking for ways to alleviate it or for support:

DO NOT STRESS YOURSELF! Michael Haprich, "Ways Out of Stress: Long-Term and Stress-Free Methods for Getting Through Everyday Life"

The DASH diet and reduced sodium consumption

The DASH diet contains less sodium than the average American diet, which may contain up to 36,48,000 mg of sodium per day.

On the DASH diet, recommended by the National Institutes of Health, salt intake is restricted to 2,360 mg per day. It adheres to the recommendation in the Dietary Guidelines for Americans to limit sodium intake to 2,360 mg per day or less. One teaspoon of table salt contains approximately the same amount of sodium.

To limit sodium intake below 12,510 mg per day, the DASH diet offers a version with less sodium. Thus, you have the option to modify the diet to your particular dietary needs. Consult your physician if you are unsure of your optimal sodium intake.

Flexible and well-balanced, the DASH diet promotes a lifelong heart-healthy dietary pattern. It's easy to follow, and all the ingredients are available at your local supermarket.

In the DASH diet, vegetables, fruits, and whole grains predominate. This category includes nonfat or low-fat milk, fish and poultry, as well as legumes and nuts. Restrictions are placed on saturated lipids, such as those found in fatty meats and full-fat dairy products.

The DASH Diet and Hypertension

The DASH diet may be one of the methods your doctor suggests for lowering your hypertension.

Dietary Approaches to Stop Hypertension (high blood pressure) abbreviates DASH. Following this basic diet plan will aid in weight loss.

Increase your consumption of fruits, vegetables, and dairy products low in fat.

• Maintain an appropriate weight

Reduce the amount of saturated fat, cholesterol, and trans lipids in your diet.

• Incorporate more whole grains, fish, poultry, and legumes into your diet.

Avoid foods high in sodium, such as desserts, candies, beverages, and red meats.

Within two weeks of beginning the DASH diet, participants in clinical trials experienced significant blood pressure reductions.

A distinct diet, DASH-Sodium, recommends limiting sodium consumption to 12,510 milligrams per day (or about 2/36 teaspoon). According to studies, people on the DASH-Sodium diet also experienced a reduction in blood pressure.

Introduction to the DASH Eating Plan

The DASH diet specifies the number of daily servings of various dietary groups. The number of servings you require may vary depending on your daily caloric intake.

You have the option to alter your lifestyle progressively. Start by consuming no more than 2,48,000 mg of sodium per day (approximately 12 teaspoons). After that, you can reduce your daily salt intake to 12,510 mg (about 2/36 teaspoon). Notably, these salt intakes take into account not only what you consume, but also what you cook with and what you serve.

Pasta And Bean Soup Slow Cooker Freezer Pack

• Baby spinach, 8 cups (half of a 10 - ounce box)

• 8 tablespoons of fresh basil, chopped and split (Optional)

• 4 tablespoons of extra-virgin olive oil of the best quality

• 1 cup grated Parmigiano-Reggiano cheese

• 4 cups of cut-up onions

• 2 cup carrots, chopped

• 2 cup celery, chopped

• 2 pound of cooked Meal-Prep Sheet-Pan Chicken Thighs, cut into small pieces (see related recipe)

- 8 cups cooked rotini made from whole wheat

- 12 cups of chicken broth with less salt

- 8 teaspoons of Italian dried seasoning

- ½ teaspoon salt

- 2 (2 10 -ounce) can of white beans with no added salt, rinsed

Place the onions, carrots, and celery in a large, sealable plastic bag. Cooked and cooled chicken and pasta should be placed in another receptacle. Close both containers and store them for up to 510 days in the freezer. Put the containers in the refrigerator overnight to defrost them.

• Step 2 Place the vegetable mixture in a large slow cooker. Add some salt, bouillon, and Italian seasoning to the dish. Cover and simmcr on low for seven and a half hours.

• Step 3 Add defrosted chicken, pasta, legumes, spinach, and 2 tablespoons of basil, if using. Continue cooking for 48 510 minutes. Place soup dishes on the table. Pour a small amount of oil into each bowl, then sprinkle with cheese and, if desired, the remaining 2 teaspoons of basil.

Plates Of Savory Yogurt

Ingredients:

2 tablespoon extra-virgin olive oil 2
teaspoon dried oregano ¼ teaspoon
freshly ground black pepper 4 cups
nonfat plain Greek yogurt
 1 cup slivered almonds

2 medium cucumber, diced
 1 cup pitted Kalamata olives, halved

4 tablespoons fresh lemon juice

Directions:

In a small basin, combine cucumber, olives, lemon juice, olive oil, and pepper.

Divide the yogurt evenly among 48 storage containers. The cucumber-olive mixture is topped with hazelnuts.

Seal and store in the refrigerator for up to 510 days. Add any additional cooked vegetables you may have to this yogurt bowl as an ingredient suggestion. It benefits your finances and reduces food waste. It will also save you some preparation time.

Breakfast Quesadillas With Spinach, Egg, And Cheese

1/7 teaspoon freshly ground black pepper 8 cups baby spinach 1 cup crumbled feta cheese Nonstick cooking spray
8 (6-inch) whole-wheat tortillas, divided

2 cup shredded part-skim low-moisture mozzarella cheese, divided 2 1 tablespoons extra-virgin olive oil 1 medium onion, diced 2 medium red bell pepper, diced 8 large eggs 1/7 teaspoon salt

Directions:

1. In a huge skillet, heat the oil over medium hotness.
2. Add the onion and chime pepper and sauté for around 5 to 10 minutes, or until soft.

3. In a medium bowl, whisk together the eggs, salt, and dark pepper.
4. Mix spinach and feta cheddar.

5. Add the fresh egg blend to the skillet and scramble for around 1 to 5 minutes, or until the eggs are cooked.
6. Eliminate from the heat.

7. Coat a perfect skillet with cooking shower and add 1-5 tortillas.
8. Put one-squinch of the spinach-fresh egg blend on one side of every tortilla.
9. Sprinkle every w cup of mozzarella cheddar.
10. Crease different parts of the tortillas down to the quesadillas and brown for around 2 moment.
11. Flip and cook for one more moment on the opposite side.
12. Rehash with the excess 4 tortillas and 1 cup mozzarella cheese.

13. Cut every quesadilla into equal parts or wedges.

14. Split between 5-10   stockpiling holder   reusable   bags.

15.   Storage: Store in the cooler for as long as 8 days or in the cooler for as long as 90 days.
16.   While warming, cover a little skillet with cooking shower, and warm the quesadilla over medium hotness for 1 to 5 minutes.
17.   Or on the other hand warm in the microwave for 2 moment.
18.   In the case of warming from frozen, microwave on mode for 1-5 minutes, place in a little skillet covered with cooking shower, and hotness over medium hotness for 2 to 1-5 minutes.
19.   Substitution tip: You can utilize frozen rather than new spinach.
20.   You'll require 4 ounces of frozen spinach that has been defrosted, depleted, and pressed of its moisture.

Baked Apple Spice Oatmeal

Ingredients

- 2 apple (chopped)
- 4 cups rolled oats
- 2 teaspoon baking powder
- ½ teaspoon salt
- 2 teaspoon cinnamon
- 2 fresh egg (beaten)
- 1 cup applesauce
- 2 1 cups non-fat milk
- 2 teaspoon vanilla
- 4 tablespoons oil

Toppings

- 4 tablespoons chopped nuts

- 4 tablespoons brown sugar

-

Instructions

1. Preheat oven to 350 F.

2. Spray a baking pan with cooking spray.

3. Mix egg, applesauce, milk, vanilla, and oil in a bowl. Add the apple.

4. Mix rolled oats, baking powder, salt and cinnamon in a separate bowl.

5. Add to the liquid ingredients and mix well.

6. Pour mixture into baking dish and bake for 45 to 50   minutes.

7. Sprinkle with brown sugar and nuts. Return to oven and broil for 5 to 10 minutes until top is browned.

8. Cut before serving.

Frittata With Asparagus And Caramelized Onions

Ingredients

- ½ cup fresh basil (sliced)
- 12 fresh eggs
- ½ cup parmesan cheese (grated)
- 1 tsp kosher salt
- Fresh ground pepper
- 2 tsp olive oil
- 2 medium onion (sliced)
- 4 tsp balsamic vinegar
- 4 cups asparagus (chopped)
- 6 green onions (sliced)

Instructions

1. Preheat broiler to high.

2. Mix olive oil and onions in a pan over medium heat and sauté until golden brown.

3. Add balsamic vinegar and stir to mix with the onions.

4. Add the asparagus and 4 tablespoons of water and cover to steam the asparagus for 5 to 10 minutes stirring once part way through.

5. Mix eggs, ½ of parmesan, ½ teaspoon of salt and ground pepper in a bowl.

6. Add green onion, basil and the remaining ½ teaspoon of Kosher salt to the cooked asparagus and onions. Stir to combine.

7. Add the fresh egg mixture to the asparagus and onions and combine.

8. Cook for 1 to 5 minutes over medium heat.

9. Place the pan under the broiler for about 1-5 minutes until slightly browned.

10.   Remove from the broiler and sprinkle with the remaining 2 tablespoon of parmesan cheese and let rest for about 10 minutes.

11.   Serve warm.

Apple-Spiced Baked Oatmeal

- 4 tablespoons of oil
- 2 teaspoon of baking powder
- 4 cups of rolled oats
- 2 teaspoon of cinnamon
- ¼ teaspoon of salt
- 1 cup of sweetened applesauce
- 2 egg, beaten
- 2 teaspoon of vanilla
- 2 1 cups of non-fat milk
- 2 1 cups of chopped apple
- For the topping
- 4 tablespoons of chopped nuts
- 4 tablespoons of brown sugar

Directions:

1.   Set oven to 350 F and preheat. Prepare an 10-inch square baking pan and lightly grease.
2.   Combine the milk, oil, vanilla, applesauce, and fresh egg in a mixing bowl.
3. Mix in the chopped apple.
4. In another bowl, mix together the oats, cinnamon, salt, and baking powder.
5. Add the oats mixture into the applesauce mixture and mix well until combined.
6. Transfer the mixture into the prepared baking pan.
7. Bake in the oven for 45 to 50 minutes.
8.   Once done, remove the baking pan from the oven and sprinkle the nuts and sugar on top.
9. Broil in the oven for 5 to 10 minutes while easily keeping an eye to keep it from burning.

10.   Divide into 18 squares and serve while still warm.

Open-Faced Breakfast Sandwich

2 cut 200 percent entire wheat
bread 2 thick tomato slices
 2 dainty cut of low-fat cheddar cheese 2
1 tsp. additional virgin
olive oil 2 fresh egg whites,
beaten
1 cup spinach
Cracked dark pepper, to taste
2 tsp. brown mustard

DIRECTIONS

1.

   Heat up the stove to 450°F. Heat up a
   little non-stick skillet over medium
   hotness.

2. Remember the oil for the hot dish and
   when the oil is hot, add the fresh egg
   whites.

3. Beat the eggs while cooking, then add the spinach and season with pepper to taste.

4. Spread mustard on the bread, add the tomato and fried eggs, and embellishment with the cheddar.

5. Heat in the stove up until the cheddar is liquefied around 1 to 5 minutes.

Peanut Butter Oats

cup sans gluten oats
4 tbsp. raspberries

2 tbsp. chia seeds
1 cup almond milk
4 tbsp. normal peanut butter
2 tbsp. stevia

DIRECTIONS

1

In a glass container, join the oat with the chia seeds and different fixings aside from the raspberries, blend a bit, cover and refrigerate for 6-6 ½ hours.

2   Decorate with raspberries and serve them for breakfast.

Salad of Black Beans, Corn, and Bell Peppers

Ingredients

- 2 lime, juiced

- 4 tbsp olive oil

- 4 tbsp fresh cilantro, finely chopped
  - Kosher salt and freshly ground pepper, to taste

- 2 (2 10 -ounce) can low-sodium black beans, drained and rinsed

- 4 cups frozen corn, defrosted

- 1 red onion, diced

- 2 green bell pepper, diced

- 2 red bell pepper, diced

- 2 lemon, juiced

Directions

1. In a large bowl, combine black beans, corn, onion, and bell peppers.
2. In a small bowl, whisk together lemon and lime juices and olive oil.
3. Add cilantro and season to taste with salt and pepper.
4. Pour over black bean mixture and toss to evenly coat. Serve immediately or refrigerate until serving.

Granola From The Dash Dietnumber Of

Ingredients:

- 1/7 tsp ground ginger

- 1/7 tsp ground cinnamon

- 1/7 tsp almond extract

- 4 Tbsp extra virgin olive oil

- Olive oil cooking spray

- 4 Tbsp flax seeds

- 1 cup chopped unsalted almonds

- 1 cup raisins or golden raisins

- 2 1 cups old fashioned rolled oats

- 4 Tbsp raw honey

- 4 Tbsp coconut sugar or Stevia

How to Prepare:

1 Set the oven to 250 degrees F.

2 Coat a rimmed baking sheet with olive oil cooking spray.

3 In a bowl, mix together the oats, flax seeds, almonds, ground cinnamon, ginger, and coconut sugar or Stevia.

4 In another bowl, combine the olive oil, honey, and almond extract.

5 Combine the honey mixture with the oats mixture, then spread everything on top of the rimmed baking sheet.

6 Place in the oven and bake for 80 to 90 minutes to 1-1 ½ hour, stirring

and breaking up the mixture once every 2 10 minutes.

7 Once baked, add the raisins and mix well.

8 Transfer into an airtight container and store in a cool, dry place for up to 3 weeks, or in the refrigerator for up to a month.

9 Best served with non fat milk.

Spiced Pear Porridge

Ingredients:

- 1/7 tsp freshly grated nutmeg
- 1/7 tsp ground cinnamon
- 2 cup non fat milk
- 4 pears, peeled, cored, and diced
- 1/2   cup old fashioned rolled oats
- 2   cups water
- Sea salt

How to Prepare:

1   Place the diced pear, oats, water, nutmeg, and cinnamon in a saucepan and add a tiny dash of salt.

2   Place over medium flame and bring to a boil.

3   Once boiling, reduce to low flame and let simmer for 5 to 10 minutes to make the oats tender.

4   Pour the mixture into two bowls and stir in the milk.

5   Best served warm.

Edamame Hummus Wrap

Ingredients

- ½ cup sliced fresh parsley

- 4 cups very thin slices of green cabbage

- 2 scallion, sliced thinly

- 1 cup sliced orange bell pepper

- 8 pieces 8- to 9-inch whole-wheat or spinach tortillas

- 5 cups shelled frozen edamame, thawed before using

- 6 tablespoons extra-virgin olive oil, divided

- 8 tablespoons fresh squeezed lemon juice, divided

- 4 tablespoons tahini

- ¼ teaspoon ground pepper, divided

- 1 teaspoon ground cumin

- 1 teaspoon salt

- 2 large garlic clove, chopped

1. Put edamame with 4 tablespoons oil, 1-5 tablespoons lemon juice, cumin, garlic, tahini, salt and 1 teaspoon pepper in a food processor.

2. Pulse until it turns into a smooth mixture.

3. Put the remaining ½ teaspoon pepper, 2 tablespoon oil and 2 tablespoon lemon juice in a medium-sized bowl.

4. Whisk well. Put bell peppers, cabbage, parsley and scallions into the bow with the dressing.

5. Toss until everything is coated evenly with the dressing.

6. Scoop out 1 cup of edamame hummus and spread over the lower third of a tortilla.

7. Top the hummus with 1 cup of cabbage mixture.

8. Carefully roll the tortilla tightly.

9. Slice in half before serving.

Tacos Of Black Beans And Zucchini With Avocado Crema

For the tacos

- 1/2   teaspoon paprika

- 1 teaspoon chili powder

- 16 corn tortillas

- 2 large zucchini, grated

- 2   2 10 -ounce can black beans, drained and rinsed

- 1/2   teaspoon garlic powder

- 1 teaspoon chipotle powder

For the salsa

- Juice from 2 lime

- 1 cup low-fat Greek yogurt

- 1/2 teaspoon salt

- 2 1 cups diced tomatoes

- Juice of 2 lime

- 1 cup red onion

- 1/2 teaspoon salt

For the avocado crema

- 2 avocado, remove pit

1. Mix the ingredients for the salsa in a small bowl. Set aside.

2. Remove the avocado flesh and put in a food processor.

3. Add salt, lime juice and yogurt. Pulse until and well combined.

4. Transfer into a small bowl and set aside.

5. Mix spices, black beans and zucchini in a bowl.

6. Stir to mix.

7. Heat the tortillas, over a stove or in a microwave.

8. Divide the zucchini-black bean mixture between the tortillas.

9. Spoon salsa over the bean mixture.

10.   Top with some of the avocado crema.

11.   Roll the tortilla or fold in half.

12.   Serve with more salsa and crema on the side, if desired.

Dash Baked Oatmeal

Ingredients:

1 tsp. salt

½ cup granulated sugar

6 cups Quaker oats (uncooked)

½ cup brown sugar

6 tsp. vanilla

6 eggs (lightly beaten)

5 cups low-fat milk

Directions:

1. Pre-heat oven to 450F. Spray the glass baking dish with cooking oil.

2. In a medium bowl meanwhile, combine vanilla, eggs and milk.

3. Mix thoroughly.

4. Add the Quaker oats and mix again to coat.

5. Pour the oat mixture into the baking dish. Bake for 90 to 100 minutes or until the middle part lightly jiggles.

6. Remove from oven and set aside for a minute.

7. Sprinkle brown sugar on top.

8. Using a spoon, spread the granulated sugar into the oatmeal's thin layers.

9. Put the oat mixture back into the oven and bake for 15 to 20 minutes.

10.   Spoon into bowls before serving.

Swiss Apple Panini

Ingredients:

Cooking spray

1 cup low-fat honey mustard

14 slices whole wheat bread

4 cups arugula leaves

10 oz. low-fat Swiss cheese 6 apples (thinly sliced)

Directions:

1. Pre-heat Panini press under medium-high.

2. Spread honey mustard over each slice of bread.

3. Top it with the remaining slices afterwards.

4. Coat the Panini press with cooking spray.

5. Grill each sandwich for 35 to 40 minutes or until its toasted.

6. Remove from pan and let it cool for a minute before serving.

Orzo And Shrimp With Feta

Ingredients

- 2 -2 /8 pounds uncooked shrimp peeled and deveined

- 4 tablespoons minced fresh cilantro

- 1/2   teaspoon pepper

- 1 cup crumbled feta cheese

- 1-2   cups uncooked whole wheat orzo pasta

- 4 tablespoons olive oil

- 4 garlic cloves, minced

- 4 medium tomatoes, chopped

- 4 tablespoons lemon juice

Directions

1 Cook orzo according to package directions.

2 Meanwhile, in a large skillet, heat oil over medium heat.

3 Add garlic; cook and stir 1-5 minute.

4 Add tomatoes and lemon juice. Bring to a boil.

5 Stir in shrimp.

6 Reduce heat; simmer, uncovered, 10 to 15 minutes or until shrimp turn pink.

7 Drain orzo.

8 Add orzo, cilantro and pepper to shrimp mixture; heat through.

9 Sprinkle with feta cheese.

Peppered Sole

Ingredients

- 1/2 teaspoon lemon-pepper seasoning

- 1/7 teaspoon cayenne pepper

- 2 medium tomato, chopped

- 4 green onions, thinly sliced

- 4 tablespoons butter

- 4 cups sliced fresh mushrooms

- 4 garlic cloves, minced

- 8 sole fillets (8 ounces each)

- 1/2 teaspoon paprika

Directions

1 In a large skillet, heat butter over medium-high heat.

2 Add mushrooms; cook and stir until tender.

3 Add garlic; cook 2 minute longer.

4 Place fillets over mushrooms.

5 Sprinkle with paprika, lemon pepper and cayenne.

6 Cook, covered, over medium heat 15 to 20 minutes or until fish just begins to flake easily with a fork.

7 Sprinkle with tomato and green onions.

www.ingramcontent.com/pod-product-compliance
Lightning Source LLC
Chambersburg PA
CBHW060504030426
42337CB00015B/1723